Fatigue syndrome

facts on treatment of chronic fatique that should be noted

Dr Walt wade

Contents

chapter1 3

introduction to chronic fatique syndron 3

Chapter2.....................................15

. Current Treatments and Management Options for Chronic Fatigue Syndrome 15

Chapter3......................................22

Debunking Myths and Misconceptions About Chronic Fatigue Syndrome...................22

The end.....................................29

chapter1

introduction to chronic fatique syndron

Chronic Fatigue Syndrome (CFS), also known as myalgic encephalomyelitis (ME), is a complex and poorly understood medical condition characterized by severe and persistent fatigue that is not relieved by rest and is not caused by any underlying medical condition. This debilitating illness affects millions of people worldwide, and yet it remains a highly stigmatized and underdiagnosed condition. The first case of what is now known as CFS was described in the 1980s, and since then, numerous studies have been conducted to investigate its causes, symptoms, and treatment options. However, despite decades of research, there is still no definitive consensus on what exactly causes CFS. This lack of understanding makes it challenging for medical professionals to diagnose and effectively treat patients, leading to confusion and frustration for those suffering from this condition. The primary symptom of CFS is severe fatigue that does not improve with rest and significantly interferes with daily activities, lasting for at least six months or longer. This fatigue is not due to overexertion, and even minimal physical or mental activity can worsen symptoms. Other common symptoms include muscle aches and pains, joint pain, headache, difficulty concentrating, memory problems, sore throat, and enlarged lymph nodes. One of the main challenges in diagnosing CFS is that its symptoms are shared by many other medical conditions, making it a diagnosis of exclusion. This means that other potential causes of fatigue, such as thyroid disorders, anemia, and autoimmune diseases, must be ruled out before a diagnosis of CFS can be made. As a result, it often takes several years and multiple doctor's visits for a person to receive a proper diagnosis, leading to delayed treatment and prolonged suffering. Aside from physical symptoms, CFS also has a significant impact on a person's mental and emotional well-being. The persistent fatigue and lack of understanding and support from others can lead to feelings of isolation, depression, and anxiety. CFS also takes a toll on a person's social life, forcing them to miss out on events and activities that they once enjoyed. All of these factors contribute to the overall negative impact of CFS on a person's quality of life. The exact causes of CFS are still unknown, but there are several theories that have been proposed by researchers and medical professionals. Some studies have suggested that viral infections, such as the Epstein-Barr virus and human herpesvirus 6, may trigger the onset of CFS in some individuals. Others believe that it may be an autoimmune disorder, where the body's immune system mistakenly attacks its tissues, leading to chronic inflammation and fatigue. Genetic predisposition is also thought to play a role in the development of CFS, as it tends to run in families. Environmental factors, such as exposure to certain toxins or stressors, may also contribute to the development of CFS in susceptible individuals. However, more research is needed to confirm these theories and fully understand the underlying cause of this complex illness. There is no definitive cure for CFS, and treatment options are focused on managing symptoms and improving quality of life. Due to the wide range of symptoms and individual differences among patients, treatment plans may vary from person to person. Some approaches may include medications for pain, sleep, and depression, as well as lifestyle changes such as dietary modifications, exercise, and stress management techniques.

Alternative therapies, such as acupuncture and cognitive-behavioral therapy, have also shown some promise in managing CFS symptoms. In recent years, there has been an increasing recognition of CFS as a legitimate medical condition, and efforts are being made to raise awareness and improve understanding of this illness. However, there is still a long way to go in terms of research, diagnosis, and effective treatment options. For those living with CFS, the day-to-day struggle with fatigue, pain, and other symptoms is an ongoing battle. However, it is vital to remember that this condition is not a sign of weakness or laziness. CFS is a complex and debilitating illness that requires patience, understanding, and support from both medical professionals and society as a whole. In conclusion, Chronic Fatigue Syndrome is a challenging and poorly understood illness that affects millions of people worldwide. Its debilitating symptoms and lack of a definitive cause make it a frustrating and often stigmatized condition. More research and awareness are needed to improve diagnosis and treatment options for those living with CFS. Until then, it is essential to show compassion and support for those affected by this chronic illness.

The Impact of Chronic Fatigue Syndrome on Daily Life

The most prominent symptom of CFS is overwhelming fatigue that is not relieved by rest and persists for at least six months. This fatigue is often described as a deep, unrelenting exhaustion that makes every task seem insurmountable. It differs from regular tiredness in that rest or sleep does not alleviate it, and pushing through the fatigue can often result in a worsened condition. This debilitating exhaustion greatly impacts daily life, as tasks that may seem ordinary to others become nearly impossible for those with CFS. One of the most significant ways that CFS affects daily life is through the impact it has on a person's ability to work or go to school. With the persistent fatigue and other symptoms, many individuals with CFS find it challenging to maintain a regular job or attend classes. This can result in significant financial strain, as well as feelings of guilt and inadequacy, as many CFS sufferers are unable to contribute to their household's income or meet their educational goals. In some cases, individuals with CFS are forced to leave their jobs or drop out of school entirely, further adding to their physical, emotional, and financial burden. Even simple daily tasks such as household chores or errands can be insurmountable for individuals with CFS. Basic activities like cooking, cleaning, or even taking a shower can leave them feeling drained and exhausted for hours or even days. This can lead to a loss of independence and reliance on others for basic needs. The physical limitations caused by CFS make it challenging for individuals to maintain a sense of normalcy in their daily lives, resulting in feelings of isolation and frustration. Moreover, the symptoms of CFS can often mimic those of other conditions, making it difficult for sufferers to receive an accurate diagnosis. This lack of understanding and recognition of the condition can lead to significant challenges in daily life, including delayed treatment and inappropriate medical care. Without proper treatment, the symptoms of CFS can worsen, further impacting a person's ability to function and perform daily tasks. CFS also has a significant impact on a person's mental health, leading to feelings of depression, anxiety, and social isolation. With the constant fatigue and inability to engage in regular activities, many CFS sufferers feel trapped in their own bodies, unable to participate in activities they once enjoyed. This can lead to a loss of self-identity and a sense of purpose, as well as feelings of frustration, anger, and hopelessness. Additionally, the lack of understanding and support from friends and family can exacerbate these feelings, further isolating the individual suffering from CFS. The financial strain and limitations on daily tasks caused by CFS have a ripple effect in a person's life. Many individuals with CFS are not able to attend social gatherings or events, leading to a decline in social connections. This, paired with the stigma attached to the condition, can leave individuals feeling excluded and misunderstood, further impacting their mental health. The lack of a definite cause or cure for CFS also contributes to the negativity surrounding the condition, as many individuals are accused of exaggerating their illness or told that it is all in their head. Furthermore, the unpredictable nature of CFS makes it challenging to plan for the future or make long-term commitments. The symptoms may come and go, making it challenging to predict when a person will have the energy to accomplish tasks, attend events, or make plans. This can lead to frustration and disappointment for both the individual with CFS and their loved ones.

Chapter2

. Current Treatments and Management Options for Chronic Fatigue Syndrome

1. Lifestyle changes One of the first steps in managing CFS is making necessary lifestyle changes to help reduce symptoms and improve overall well-being. These changes may include reducing stress, improving sleep hygiene, and incorporating regular exercise into one's routine. Stress management techniques such as yoga, meditation, and deep breathing exercises can help alleviate the mental and physical strain associated with CFS. Developing healthy sleep habits, such as establishing a regular bedtime routine

and avoiding caffeine and electronics before bed, can improve the quality and quantity of sleep. Regular exercise, such as low-impact activities like walking or swimming, can also improve symptoms of CFS and boost energy levels. 2. Cognitive Behavioral Therapy (CBT) Cognitive Behavioral Therapy (CBT) is a commonly used treatment for CFS as it helps patients change their thoughts and behaviors to improve their ability to cope with their condition. This form of therapy helps patients develop practical and useful coping strategies, manage stress, and reduce the negative impact of CFS on their daily lives. CBT may also address any underlying psychological factors that may contribute to CFS symptoms, such as anxiety or depression. 3. Graded Exercise Therapy (GET) Graded Exercise Therapy (GET) is a treatment approach that involves gradually increasing physical activity levels to improve overall fitness and reduce CFS symptoms. This therapy is based on the idea that gradual and controlled exercise can help improve physical and mental functioning in individuals with CFS. A therapist will create a personalized exercise program for each patient, taking into account their current level of fitness and ability. Patients are encouraged to slowly and gradually increase their activity levels over time, with close monitoring by a healthcare professional to avoid exacerbating symptoms. 4. Medications There is no specific medication approved for the treatment of CFS. However, some drugs may be prescribed to help alleviate certain symptoms of the condition. These may include: - Pain relievers: Non-steroidal anti-inflammatory drugs (NSAIDs) like ibuprofen may help reduce pain and inflammation associated with CFS. - Antidepressants: Low doses of certain antidepressants, such as tricyclic antidepressants or selective serotonin reuptake inhibitors (SSRIs), may be prescribed to help reduce fatigue, pain, and improve sleep in individuals with CFS. - Sleep aids: In cases where improving sleep through lifestyle changes is not effective, a doctor may prescribe sleep aids to help individuals with CFS get the rest they need. 5.

Nutritional Supplements Some individuals with CFS may benefit from taking certain nutritional supplements to address any nutrient deficiencies and improve overall health. Common supplements used in the treatment of CFS include: - Vitamin B12: This nutrient is essential for energy production and may help reduce fatigue in individuals with CFS. - Vitamin D: Studies have shown that individuals with CFS often have low levels of vitamin D, which plays a crucial role in immune function and may help alleviate symptoms. - Magnesium: Some individuals with CFS may have low levels of magnesium, which has been linked to fatigue and muscle weakness. Supplementing with magnesium may help improve energy levels. 6. Alternative Therapies Some individuals with CFS may seek relief from their symptoms through alternative therapies. While there is limited scientific evidence to support the effectiveness of these treatments, they may provide some relief for certain individuals. Some common alternative therapies used in the management of CFS include: - Acupuncture: This traditional Chinese therapy involves inserting thin needles into specific points in the body to improve energy flow and potentially alleviate symptoms. - Massage therapy: Incorporating regular massage sessions may help reduce pain and stiffness often experienced by individuals with CFS. - Herbal remedies: Certain herbs, such as ginseng and ashwagandha, may help improve energy levels and reduce fatigue in individuals with CFS. It is important to note that alternative therapies should be used with caution and under the supervision of a healthcare professional, as they may interact with prescribed medications or have potential side effects.

.

Chapter3

Debunking Myths and Misconceptions About Chronic Fatigue Syndrome

Myth 1: Chronic Fatigue Syndrome is not a real illness. One of the most damaging myths surrounding CFS is that it is not a real illness and that sufferers are simply lazy or depressed. This misconception has been perpetuated by the lack of understanding and awareness about the condition. However, extensive research has been done on CFS, and it has been recognized as a legitimate medical condition by organizations such as the World Health Organization and the Center for Disease Control and Prevention. CFS is a complex and multifaceted illness that affects various systems in the body, including the immune, neurological, and endocrine systems. The symptoms of CFS are very real and can significantly impact a person's daily life. Not only does this myth invalidate the experiences of those suffering from CFS, but it also prevents individuals from seeking the necessary medical help and support. Myth 2: Chronic Fatigue Syndrome only affects women. Another common myth about CFS is that it only affects women. While it is true that the majority of CFS patients are women, this does not mean that men cannot develop the condition. Studies have shown that the ratio between female and male CFS patients is around 2:1, meaning that there are significant numbers of men affected by this illness. The reason for this gender imbalance is not entirely understood, but it could be due to societal expectations and stereotypes. Men are often expected to be strong and resilient, making it harder for them to acknowledge and seek help for a condition that can leave them feeling weak and fatigued. Myth 3: Everyone with CFS experiences the same symptoms. CFS is a heterogeneous condition, meaning that its symptoms and severity can vary from person to person. While the main symptom of CFS is persistent fatigue, individuals with the condition can experience a wide range of symptoms, including muscle pain, joint pain, headaches, insomnia, and cognitive difficulties. Some people may have mild symptoms that allow them to continue with their daily activities, while others may be bedridden and unable to work or even leave their homes. The severity and combination of symptoms also vary throughout the course of the illness, making it challenging to diagnose and treat. Myth 4: Chronic Fatigue Syndrome is caused by a lack of exercise. There is a popular misconception that CFS is caused by a lack of exercise, and that sufferers would feel better if they just pushed through their fatigue and exercised more. However, exercise intolerance is a defining feature of CFS, and exertion can often make symptoms worse. The exact cause of CFS is still unknown, but research suggests that it could be triggered by a combination of factors, including viral infections, genetic predisposition, and environmental factors. It is essential for CFS patients to listen to their bodies and not push themselves beyond their limits, as this can lead to a worsening of symptoms and even relapse. Myth 5: There is a cure for Chronic Fatigue Syndrome. There is currently no cure for CFS, and while treatments can help alleviate some symptoms, they do not work for everyone. This has led to the misconception that CFS is not a legitimate illness, or that sufferers are not trying hard enough to get better. The reality is that CFS is a chronic condition, and managing its symptoms is an ongoing process. People with CFS often have to learn to adapt their lifestyles and daily routines to manage their symptoms and conserve their energy. This involves pacing themselves, setting realistic expectations, and practicing self-care. Myth 6: Chronic Fatigue Syndrome is just extreme tiredness. While fatigue is the most prominent symptom of CFS, it is not the same as just feeling tired. Fatigue in CFS is often described as a debilitating and overwhelming exhaustion that does not improve with rest. It is also not the result of physical or mental exertion, and can be accompanied by other symptoms such as brain fog, muscle pain, and flu-like symptoms. This myth can be particularly damaging as it downplays the severity of CFS and can prevent individuals from seeking proper medical help and support. Myth 7: Chronic Fatigue Syndrome is a mental illness. CFS is a complex medical condition that affects the body physically, and while mental health can play a role, it is not the cause of the illness. The symptoms of CFS can often lead to mental health problems such as depression and anxiety, but they are not the primary cause of the condition. Furthermore, the suggestion that CFS is a mental illness only adds to the stigma and can prevent individuals from receiving the medical care and support they need

The end